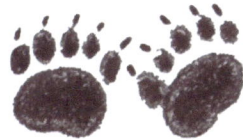

Growing Self-Esteem through Yoga

Helping children reach their

highest potential

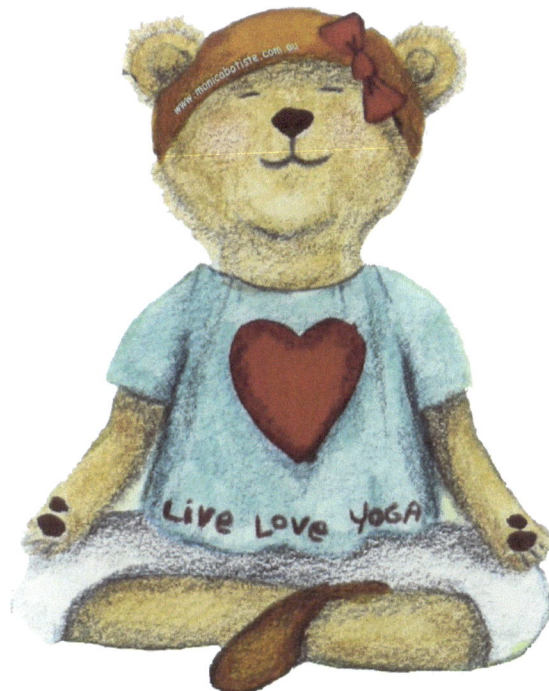

Monica Batiste

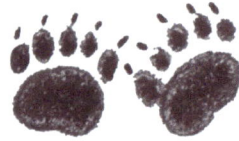

"Character isn't just about doing the right thing in an ethical sense; it is about doing our best work. If that is true, then character education isn't about helping kids get along; it is also about teaching them to work hard, develop their talents, and aspire to excellence in every area of endeavor"
Lickona & Davidson 2005, p. 573

Table of Contents

What is Emotional Intelligence?

Emotional Intelligence (EI) is the capacity to recognise your emotions, to have the ability to make healthy choices based on those emotions, and the resilience or intelligence to keep growing in a positive way.

Emotional Intelligence is a key factor for a successful and happy life

Emotionally intelligent children communicate effectively with each other, giving them an advantage in achieving their goals, and at the same time supporting the emotional needs of others.

Emotionally intelligent children don't depend on others to solve their problems, and they accept personal responsibility for how they feel.

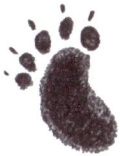

Emotional Intelligence acknowledges that all feelings are valid, even the angry ones; it is what you choose to do with those emotions that builds emotional intelligence.

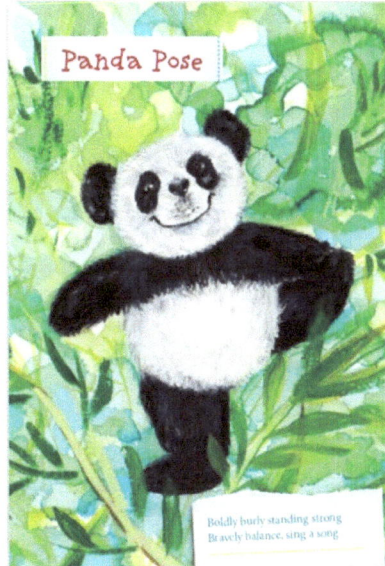

Panda Pose

Boldly burly standing strong
Bravely balance, sing a song

Panda pose helps children build confidence.

What is Yoga?

Yoga is a combination of postures and lifestyle. There are many postures practised in yoga which support strength and flexibility, but the greatest aspect of yoga is its ability to develop mindfulness and character.

The yoga philosophy is to love and accept yourself and others, just as you are. Yoga encourages non- judgment, peace, mindfulness, and caring for others. Each posture in yoga is designed to support the emotional connection to self and others. For instance, your class may be doing yoga, and in the last few minutes move into peaceful pose. There may be a child in your class that does not usually experience peace, but for a few moments experiences peace. He or she has an opportunity to 'wire' peace into their nervous system. Through persistent acknowledgement each time the child demonstrates peace (if only for a moment) the self-belief of peace grows stronger. There will come a time when this child knows what peace is, how to get there, what it feels like, and will acquire the ability to self-regulate to peace.

Each yoga posture has many virtues, and each virtue can be developed through yoga. My books and articles are focused on how to practise simple and fun yoga postures, and how to acknowledge the character benefits of each one.

Smart yoga including *Brain Gym* supports brain development through relaxing the brain and opening right and left brain hemispheres.

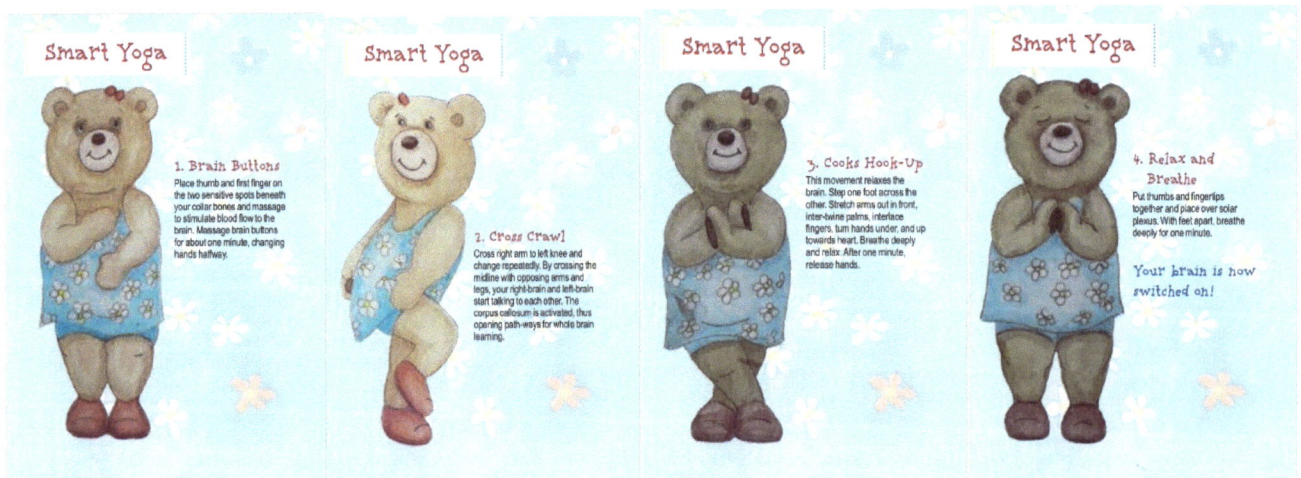

Smart Yoga from 'Yoga Bear Posture Cards'

Character development doesn't have to be boring or serious – many postures are noisy and fun. *Lion pose* for example, includes a loud roar! Children love it. On a physical level *Lion pose* improves knee flexibility, but on an emotional level, *Lion pose* releases the voice, and supports a timid child into speaking up.

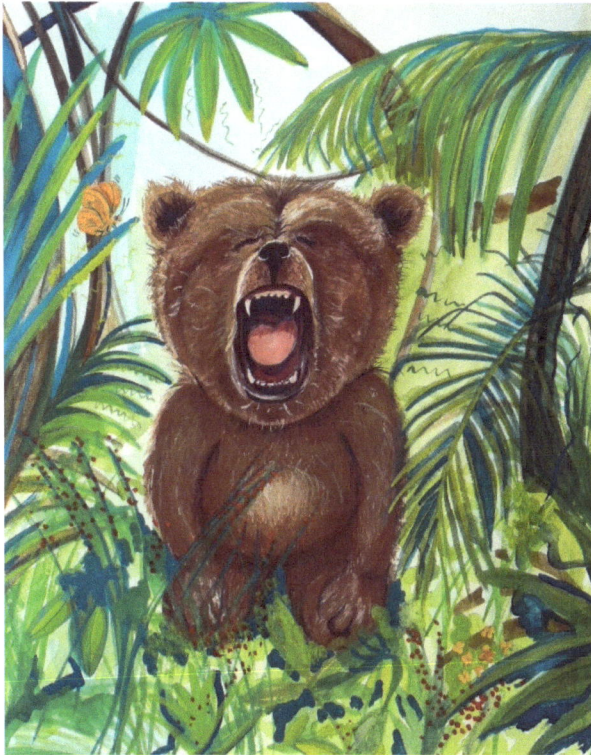

Lion Pose

Lion Pose helps clear the throat and release the voice. If a child needsto develop assertiveness, or has been through a difficult situation, *Lion Pose* gives them back their voice and can unblock emotional energy held in the throat.

It's also lots of fun and one of the children's favourites.

Virtues Developed Assertiveness, confidence, letting go of 'stuff'. To do *Lion Pose*, begin in *Hero's Pose*.

How to do Lion Pose

From *Hero's Pose,* place hands on knees, or on the floor with fingertips towards knees and forearms facing front. Open mouth wide, stick out tongue and roar like a lion. Repeat three times.

Hero's Pose

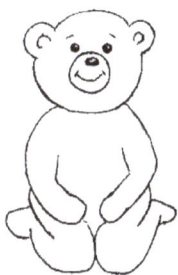

Kneel on floor with hands resting on thighs. Allow feet to 'wrap around' thigh rather than opening to side. If knees are uncomfortable, sit cross-legged or open-legged.

Benefits of Hero's Pose

Hero's Pose helps to stretch thighs and promotes knee flexibility.

I was teaching a new class and mentioned the benefits of *Lion pose*. Their teacher said, *'Well that's amazing, because the two children who refused to do Lion pose are my two timid children.'*

Yoga offers tools to strengthen and stretch the whole body, to de-stress and increase calm, peace and happiness. The mindfulness and self-acceptance practised through yoga improves emotional strength, resilience and self-esteem. Meditation raises immunity, promotes inner peace and self-love.

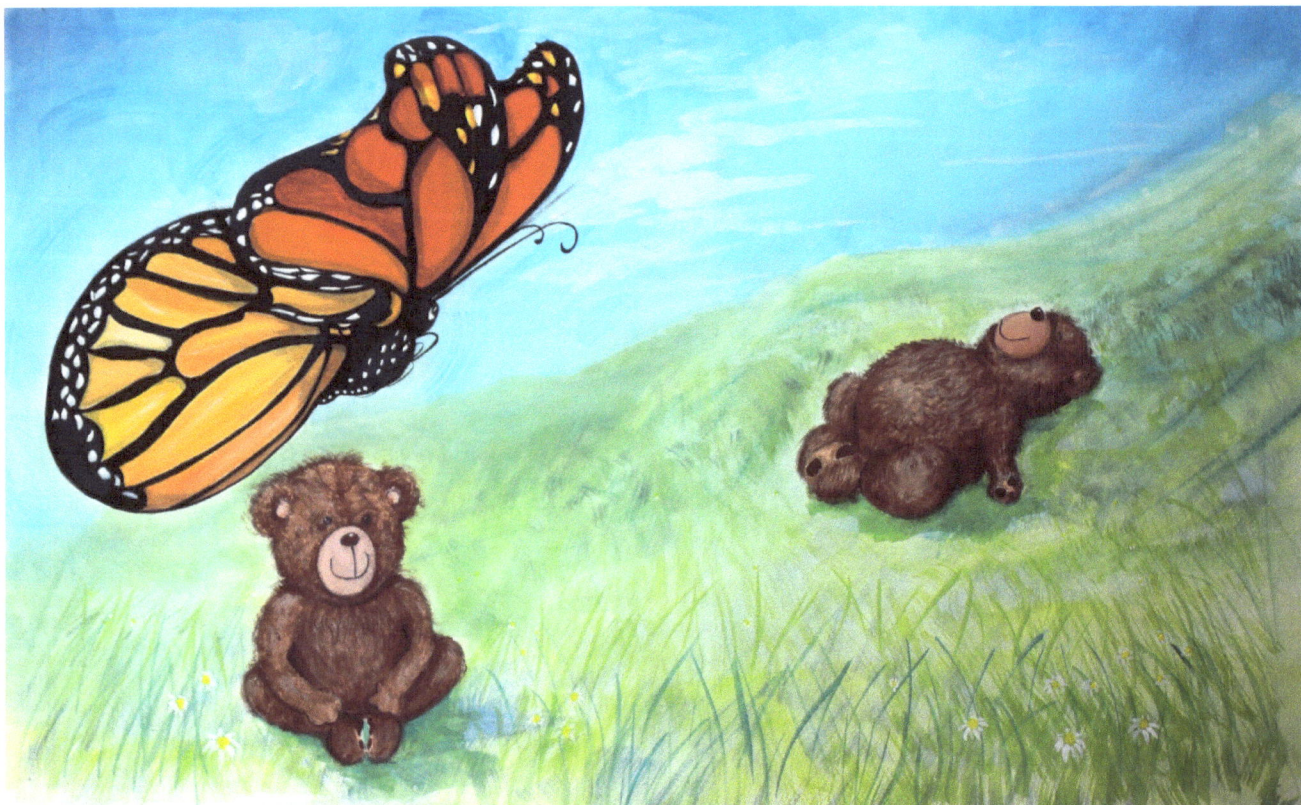

Resting Butterfly helps children find trust and calm. From *Yoga for Little Bears*

Yoga is there for the long term – it isn't something you do once and it's done. It's something that can be practised for a handful of minutes each day to maintain a high level of physical and emotional development, that will support you for life's entire journey.

The benefits derived through yoga can be drawn on every day, allowing all who practise it to experience a more loving and joyful life.

Yoga is an extension of life's moments. During yoga all virtues can be acknowledged, for each posture calls a child to a virtue, and virtues grow emotional intelligence.

Children have a natural ability to love and accept themselves, and yoga helps bring out this natural expression

Every time you name a virtue, the virtue within that child grows.

You can find virtues in every posture; for instance during *Meditation; Child's pose* or *Resting butterfly* (even if it's a few seconds), you can acknowledge your child for peacefulness. During *Tree pose* you can acknowledge focus. During *Warrior poses* you can acknowledge courage. In *Cat pose*, you can acknowledge flexibility.

Acknowledgment starts right here, wherever you are, and when you acknowledge virtues during everyday life, you see the transformation of your child's self esteem.

When your child makes the connection that they can self regulate their emotions they will thrive.

As children grow self-esteem and take charge of how they feel, they will have the resilience to make positive choices for their wellbeing.

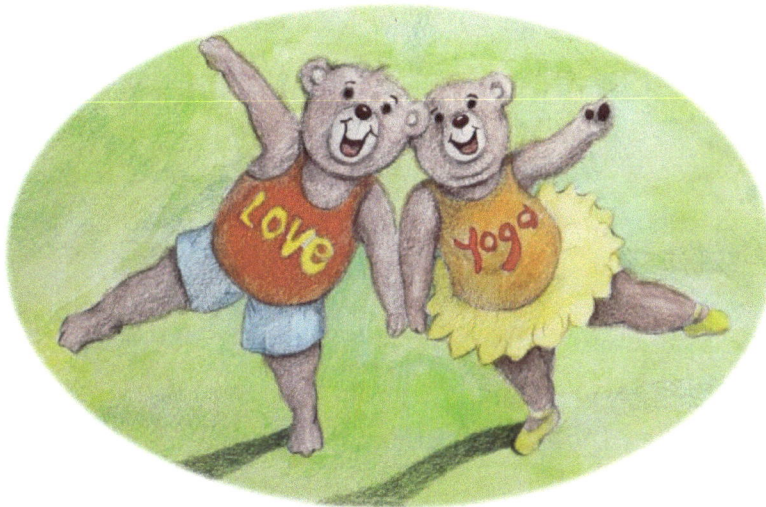

Constellation of Stars supports children to learn co-operation, balance, focus and team spirit. It also helps with connection to community. From *Yoga for Little Bears.*

Resilience is important because the higher the resilience, the easier it is for your child to recover from setbacks.

For instance when someone fails an exam, is fired or rejected, the first response may be disappointment, but how that person feels about themselves determines what they do next, and how quickly they recover.

An emotionally intelligent child with high self- esteem will acknowledge how they feel, and support themselves in a healthy way. They will understand that it hurts, know this hurt will eventually pass, not blame themselves, and as the hurt subsides, they will resume actions to achieve their goals. They will still believe in themselves.

The low self-esteem child feels defeated. They might see this as another piece of evidence that they are a failure; that they cannot achieve, and this experience might be their fault. They are likely to feel powerless and helpless, and use negative words to describe their situation. They may not try again because, 'What would be the point?'

Without emotional intelligence, children cannot successfully move through pain or overcome difficulty.

Without resilience, children may turn to sulking, anger or depression. They might permanently change the way they deal with life in order to resist the chances of being rejected in the future.

A teenage child or adult may take abuse substances to overcome the pain of 'failure'.

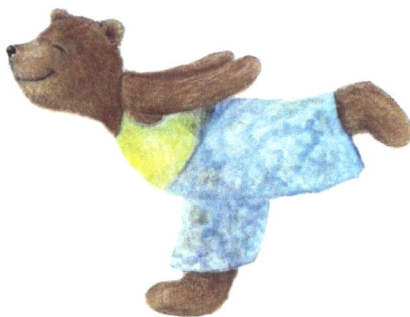

Seagull pose helps children develop balance, confidence and achievement.

The emotionally intelligent child has skills and tools to resolve and move through all situations, good and bad. Children learn this through the adults around them reflecting who they are. Role modelling positive behaviour and acknowledging virtues is a powerful tool for healing and growth.

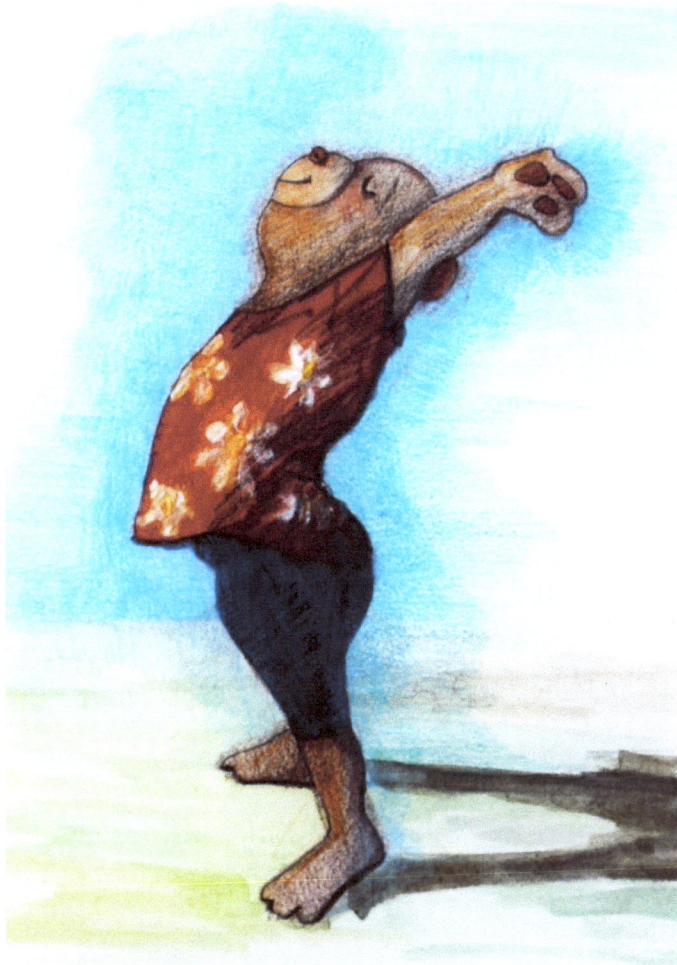

Victory pose

Victory pose is a Winner's pose. It's the posture you take when youhave won. It's how you feel when you know that you are proud ofyour achievements. Victory pose can be practiced everyday during a visualization of achievement. The winning vibe doesn't have to be about one person winning – it's about everyone winning. You can win yourown self-esteem. You can win by achieving that goal. You can win by seeing yourself as someone you love, care about and win about. You are awesome. Just as you are. You ARE a WINNER!

Virtues Developed

Self-belief, flexibility, open-heart, confidence, motivation.

How to do Victory pose

Stand strong; step one foot out to the side. Feet comfortable. Breathe in, open arms and lift up to the sky. Breath out, reach back, and face the sky. Tummy pressed in to protect spine.

Breathe deeply and feel excited about yourself. You are a WINNER! Shout HOORAY!!
Visualise yourself in that winning circle, with your winning friends, happy, smiling, laughing CELEBRATE!!
Everyone is a winner. Everyone! No matter the score, no matter the experience, everyone wins. Imagine this. Imagine you are all winners. Believe in yourself; believe in your family, Believe in your friends. You can do it. You are already doing it.

Congratulations!

The Five Aspects of Emotional Intelligence

Self-awareness, self-regulation, motivation, empathy and social skills.

Self-Awareness

Self-awareness is the ability to recognise emotions, moods and their effect on self and others. With self-awareness a child is more likely to self-assess strengths and limits, and build lateral thinking, resilience, confidence and self-worth.

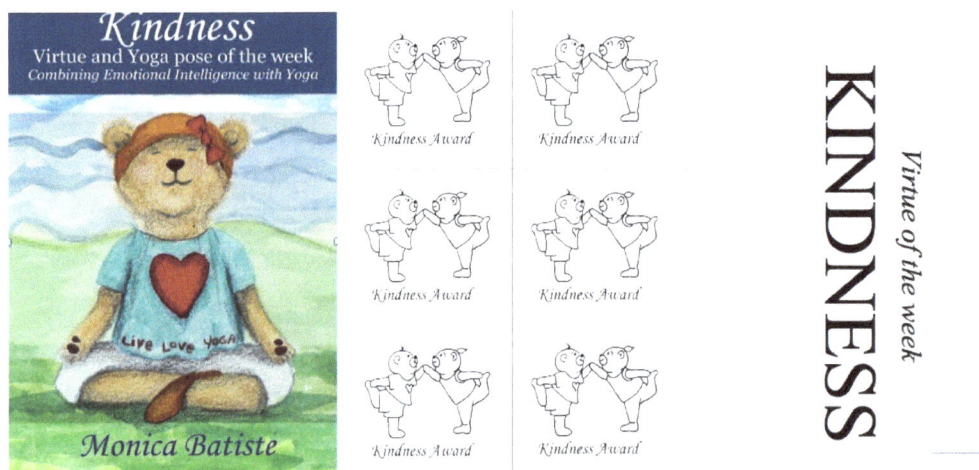

Kindness eBook from Virtue and Yoga pose of the week

Yoga helps children understand how they feel through introspection during postures. Postures reflect emotions and virtues. For example, a child that is insecure will usually reflect this through a slumped posture. Encouraging the upright posture of *Mountain pose* helps the child experience confidence. When standing tall, strong and proud in *Mountain pose*, you can acknowledge confidence, allowing the child's confidence to grow, and this will be used later in real-life situations. Being confident in yoga leads to confidence in life.

Virtues are named with each posture in my resources to help children identify and develop their self- awareness.

Yoga supports self-awareness by offering the opportunity to understand and express feelings, and the space to release when needed.

Self-Regulation

Self-regulation is the art of recognising emotions and acting on them in an appropriate way.

By teaching children to observe and name feelings (during yoga or at any time), children learn to recognise and address feelings. By showing children how to release stress through yoga, they become aware of their ability to self-regulate.

When virtues are acknowledged, children discover their moral character and use this information to regulate behaviour.

For example, when you acknowledge trust in a child, the child learns they are trustworthy, and internalise this by trusting themselves to achieve their goals.

When a child is acknowledged for assertiveness or resilience, they are more likely to initiate activities (assertiveness) and bounce back from setbacks (resilience).

During yoga, remind children that each posture is an opportunity to accept themselves 'just as they are'. Teaching self-acceptance (through words and role-modelling) gives children permission to be themselves, which builds the confidence to try new things. When people are encouraged to love and accept themselves just as they are, they flourish in a positive and productive way.

Self-regulation for the emotionally intelligent child means knowing how they feel and using these feelings to guide their behaviour for positive and healthy outcomes.

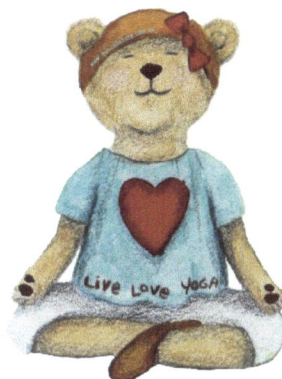

Meditation from *Yoga for Little Bears*

Meditation grows introspection, and offers a tool to find peace, no matter what, or where you are.

Meditation supports brain development by switching off stress, and increasing calm, peace, endorphins, and immunity.

Self-reflection supports self-regulation

Self-reflection grows when feelings are recognised. Support this by naming feelings: 'I can see you are angry/sad/frustrated/afraid (Name) and that is okay. How can we release this feeling so that you feel better?'

'I can see your happiness/joy/ peacefulness/confidence (Name).'

All feelings are okay; it's what you do with them that matters.

Every time you name a feeling for a child, you help them build their reservoir of emotional intelligence and their ability to relate, empathise, and grow.

Motivation

High emotional intelligence means knowing how you feel and choosing behaviour for a positive outcome

Motivation is the ability to use emotions to guide or facilitate the achievement of goals.

Motivated children have the desire to improve and do their best without the fear of making a mistake. Motivated children feel confident to align their goals with other people and have the ability to work well in a team. Motivation inspires optimism that 'all will be well'. If an emotionally intelligent child fails to achieve a goal, rather than feeling hopeless the child acknowledges their disappointment, but continues to set goals because they believe in themselves.

When motivation is high, children believe they can achieve their goals. When motivation is low, children don't believe they can achieve their goals and are reluctant to try (because failure is

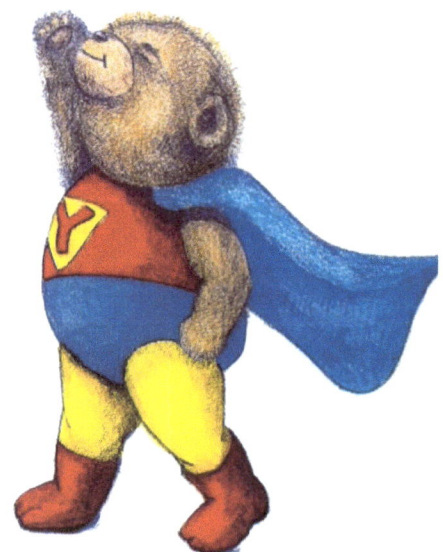

painful). The best remedy for low motivation is to build confidence and trust in the ability to achieve. This is built through many observations of positive acknowledgment.

When a child has self-belief, they retain self-respect and self-love even during setbacks.

Resilience is the gold medal for motivation

When Thomas Edison was inventing the light bulb, it took many experiments before he achieved his goal. He said, 'I have not failed. I've just found 10,000 ways that won't work.' When Olympic medallists go to the games, their goal is to do their personal best, so even if they don't achieve their ultimate goal of a gold medal, they have still won. This is an empowering attitude.

Yoga encourages motivation, as children will always achieve a yoga posture.

There is no right or wrong in yoga as all postures can be modified to suit the individual. Yoga can be practised in a wheelchair, standing or sitting; postures can work around injuries or disabilities. If a child is unable to do any of the postures, invite them to sit with the class in mindful observation, and take deep breaths. Mindful observation in yoga is a joyful way to teach 'being present', which calms and relaxes the brain.

Daily success in yoga leads to the confidence to try new things and a positive attitude for life.

The benefits of yoga are transferable. For example, when I went scuba diving for the first time, I knew I could pull myself into a boat because I was strong from yoga. I knew I could regulate my breathing through my experience with meditation. I knew I could calm myself when fear was knocking, because I had learned calming techniques through yoga.

Motivation is fuel for great achievement.

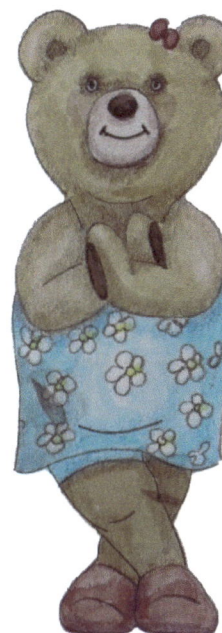

Empathy

Empathy is the ability to be aware of and take appropriate action regarding other people's feelings, needs and concerns.

Empathy is an important skill as it prevents teasing, promotes understanding, and creates unity amongst all.

When children realise that other people feel the same emotions as themselves, they develop compassion.

Yoga encourages observation of self during postures. Ask questions like 'How does this posture make you feel?' and 'How does this posture change your feelings from anger/ frustration/boredom to a better feeling?'

Using self-observation in yoga develops observation of others. The empathetic child is aware of how others are feeling and feels motivated to address it. 'Are you crying?' they might ask. 'Can I get you a tissue? A hug?'

Paired yoga supports empathy because observation of others is necessary for collaboration. Constellation of Stars pose will provide this opportunity, and the laughter that usually follows helps consolidate the good feeling of supporting others.

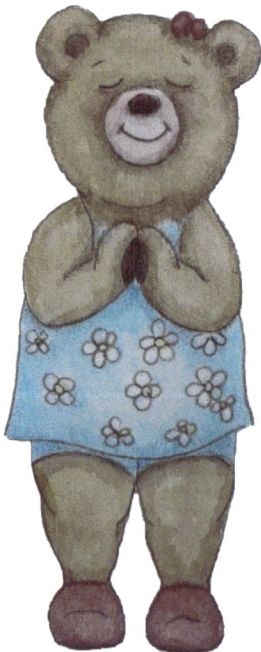

Other poses that lend themselves to pairs are Dancer's pose (holding hands), Gum-Tree pose (side by side, inner arms around each other and outer hands reaching over head like a tree branch), and Tail-balancing pose (feet touch). Have fun, invent ways to pair and support each other during yoga.

As children learn to support one another, empathy develops.

Gum Tree pose

Growing kindness for the environment by creating empathy - *Gum Tree* pose supports a child's ability to empathise, strengthen, balance, and focus. By encouraging children to imagine they are a tree; children learn to tune into others. When a child 'becomes' the tree, they grow empathy and caring for something outside themselves. Once a child has an emotional connection, they will naturally extend kindness and protection.

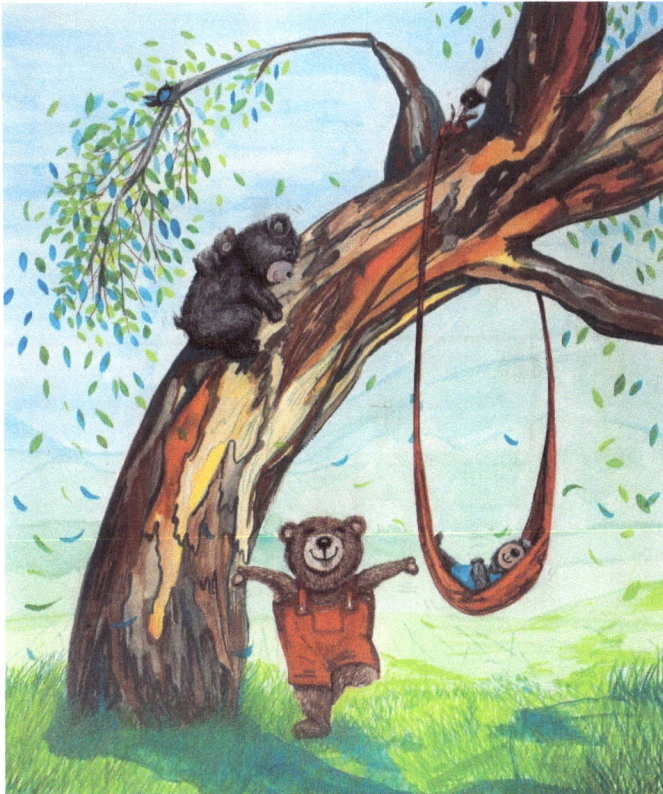

Gum Tree Pose

Gum Tree Pose helps children stay focused and calm. It improves co- ordination, core strength and balance. Practise *Gum Tree Pose* when children are scattered and need to re-focus. This is a challenging but fun exercise which will boost self-esteem.

Gum Tree Pose promotes body awareness, kinaesthetic intelligence and spatial awareness.

Virtues Developed

Focus, clarity, mindfulness, groundedness.

How to do Gum Tree Pose

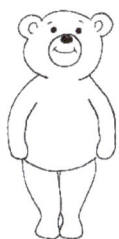
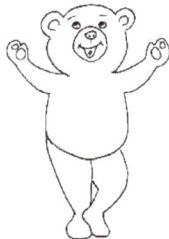
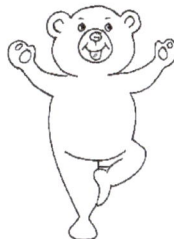

Mountain Pose   *Option 1*   *Option 2*

Start in *Mountain Pose.* Lengthen spine, tuck in tailbone, relax shoulders. Keep core strong and stay focused on one spot to help with balance. Breathe deeply. Stand on one leg and rest the other foot in front (option 1), or on the leg like a stork (option 2). Bring hands together in prayer position in front of heart or raise them above head or open them out.

'Imagine you are a beautiful tree, grounded to the earth and as high as the sky' place your hands to the heart and take another breath. 'Grow into a beautiful tree' as you grow up to the sky. 'Open your arms and pretend they are branches. Sway in the wind… side to side… around your trunk… I see your flexibility, and strength. What kind of tree are you? Can you visualize green leaves and strong branches? Are there any animals living in your tree? Can you see any birds? Or children?'

Acknowledge children for the virtues you saw and how you saw them. For example;
'Christopher I saw how gentle you were with the parrot that landed on your branch.' 'Amy I saw your imagination when you touched the clouds.'
'Paulus I saw your creativity when you decided to extend your branches.'

After a minute or so, changes sides and be a Gum tree on the other leg.

Social Skills

When you have strong social skills, you are adept at communicating your needs, and adept at eliciting desired responses from others.

The social networker can influence others towards a common goal. A strong leader has strong social skills; they know how to influence, motivate and encourage others, and have the skills to negotiate and resolve conflict.

Social skills build bonds with friends and colleagues. The social networker has empathy to offer support, guidance or correction when needed, and the intelligence to recognise the emotional or sensory language of others in order to communicate in the method that is suitable.

Yoga improves social skills as it builds the child's ability to communicate, assert their needs, and feel confident within themselves. This encourages children to take risks and form bonds with others for mutual outcomes. Partner work helps children experience support from another.

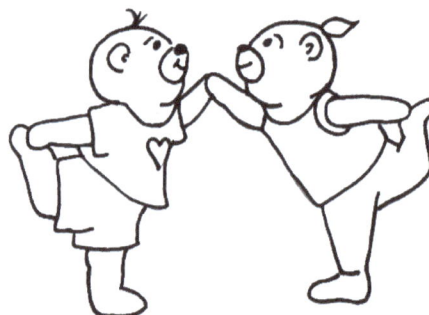

Dancer's pose with a friend

Self-Esteem

Self-esteem is how you feel about yourself.

High self-esteem means having positive beliefs and expectations about self. Low self-esteem means having negative and low expectations about self. Self-esteem can be improved through positive acknowledgment and support of students' attributes.

Friendship pose creates unity

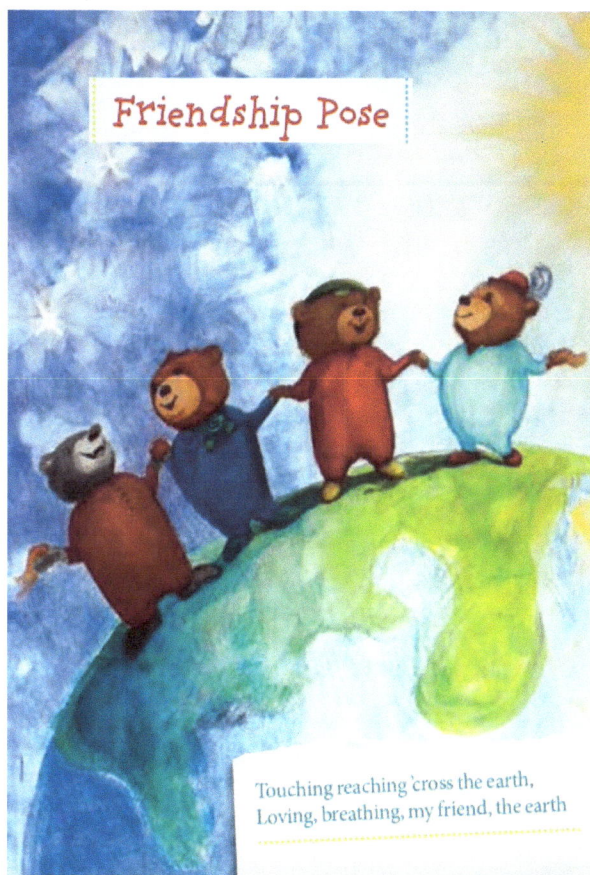

Friendship Pose

Touching reaching 'cross the earth,
Loving, breathing, my friend, the earth

Friendship Pose

Friendship is the glue that keeps us together. Where would we be without our friends? Learning to love and accept ourselves just as we are, helps us to love and accept others just as they are. We can't change another, but we can change ourselves. The more we grow and are kind to ourselves, the more we are kind to each other. Pain doesn't motivate change like happiness does. If you want to change yourself, or help a friend change, use positive language and acknowledge virtues to create loving and harmonious relationships with others.

Forgive yourself when you make a mistake, and forgive others when they make a mistake. Doing this will help you keep peace and happiness in your heart.

The better you treat yourself, the better you treat others. Good friendship begins with loving yourself.Become friends with yourself, and allow your love to shine.

Virtues Developed

Friendliness, unity, joy, happiness, compassion.

How to do Friendship Pose

Hold hands, look into each other's eyes and breathe. As thoughts come to mind, let them go, look for the love and acceptance you inherently hold for one another. This only takes a few minutes and will support any relationship to bond more deeply.

Yoga improves Emotional Intelligence by offering a space where body language reflects emotional language and by improving the body, the mind follows.

Using yoga as the tool for personal transformation is a loving, healthy, peaceful and honourable way to improve self-esteem in yourself, your family, your community and the world.

Loving the self leads to loving others.

If you are looking after you, your child will copy that. If you are loving yourself, your child will love themselves. If you are demonstrating kindness and caring towards yourself, then so will your child.

It's all about you. Love, honour and accept yourself right now, and move forward with gentleness and kindness to demonstrate emotional intelligence to your child.

Acknowledge your own successes and achievements, no matter how small, and you will automatically do this with your child, and he or she will automatically do it for themselves and others.

Yoga is an opportunity to practise virtues, acknowledgment and acceptance, because yoga postures exemplify emotions and virtues.

A student's self-talk is a strong indicator of self- esteem. For instance, 'I can't do this posture' usually means 'I don't have faith in myself ', and 'This is too hard' usually means 'Life is hard and I am afraid to try'.

Other indicators of self-esteem during yoga are pushing into postures because 'they must achieve'. This means, 'I will push myself into doing things I don't want to do even if it hurts me'.

As you notice the struggle, use this as your guide for improvement. Say things like 'There is no right or wrong; there is no need to push; just relax and allow the posture (and life) to come to you. Let go and trust that you (and the world) will support you'.

Acknowledge peaceful and self-accepting moments to show your students that life is easier if you can accept where you are in this moment.

By improving self-talk, self-esteem and communication improve.

Yoga improves self-esteem by mirroring desired virtues. Warrior poses reflect assertiveness. *Child's Pose* reflects acceptance and humility (being humble). *Lion Pose*, *Noisy Gorilla* and *Woodchopper* improve the ability to 'speak up'. *Dancer's Pose* improves grace and confidence. Virtues developed through the physical body become a part of the emotional body. All emotional experiences become part of the physical body and its shape and posture. It is all interconnected.

When you are true of purpose, in mind, body and spirit, you move with confidence and joy. When you open your heart to love, you experience freedom and spontaneity.

Balance your yoga practice with heart opening, nurturing, assertive and passive postures to help children have the healthy experience of all emotions.

All emotions are okay – because they help us see who and where we are.

You start on the mat because it's easier there; it's more obvious there. Then you move it into your life.

During postures and during the day, acknowledge virtues and allow your child to develop into the fullness of who they truly are.

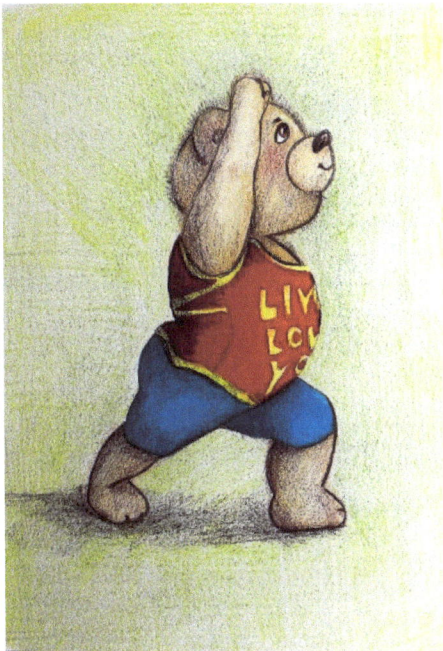

Thank you for reviewing my free resource. Please follow me to see more of my updates on character development through yoga, art, and mindfulness. If you could take the time to review my work, I'd appreciate it. If you have suggestions on how I can improve, I would appreciate that too. Thank you for your time.

Warrior one to grow confidence,

courage, and strength.

Virtues and Yoga

Acceptance
Agility
Ambition
Assertive
Attention
Awareness
Balance
Benevolence
Brave
Caring
Charity
Clarity
Cleanliness
Commitment
Compassion
Communication
Confidence
Concentration
Considerate
Consistent
Co-operation
Courage
Courtesy
Creativity
Curiosity
Dependability
Detachment
Determination
Dedication
Decisiveness
Desire

Discernment
Discretion
Discipline
Divergent thinking
Empathy
Energy
Enthusiasm
Ethics
Eloquence
Excellence
Expand comfort-zone
Faith
Flexibility
Focus
Forgiveness
Friendliness
Friendship
Fun
Generosity
Gentleness
Grace
Gratitude
Grounded
Happiness
Harmony
Health
Heroic
Holistic
Helpful
Honest
Honour

Hope
Humour
Imagination
Integrity
Initiative
Idealism
Innocence
Intuition
Joyful
Justice
Jovial
Kindness
Leadership
Letting-go
Love
Loyalty
Manners
Meditation
Mercy
Moderation
Modesty
Motivation
Negotiation
Open-Heart
Optimism
Orderliness
Patience
Peacefulness
Perseverance
Playful
Positive
Practical

Purposefulness
Reliability
Reparation
Resilience
Respect
Responsibility
Reverence
Self-Awareness
Self-Care
Self-Confidence
Self-Discipline
Self-Esteem
Self-love
Self-Reliance
Self-Respect
Self-Regulation
Service
Social-Skills
Spiritual
Steadfast
Strength
Sincerity
Tact
Tenderness
Thankfulness
Tolerance
Trust
Truthfulness
Unity
Understanding
Visionary
Wisdom
Zealous

Virtue and Yoga pose of the week
www.monicabatiste.com.au

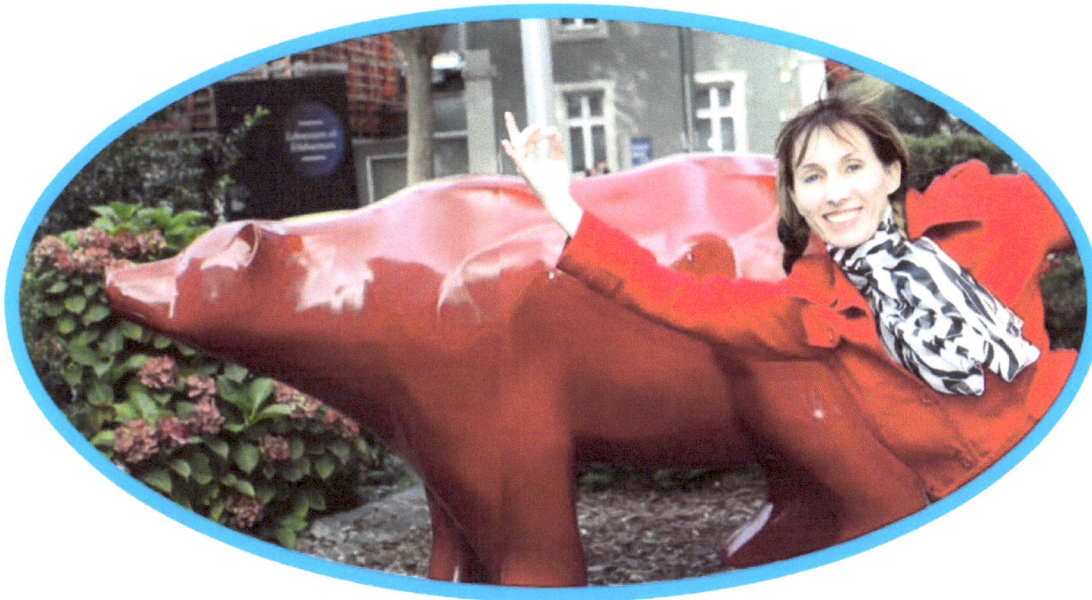

About Monica Batiste

Author, artist and yoga teacher. Monica has worked in the health and fitness industry for over 30 years. For the past 10 years her focus has been on developing emotional intelligence through yoga.

Monica teaches classes at Suttons beach in Redcliffe. She offers professional development for teachers to bring yoga into their classroom, and has published several books on yoga and emotional intelligence including strategies for anti-bullying.

As a trained artist Monica brings unique illustrations to her work that demonstrate her love of children and personal development. Her mission is to bring positive change and hope. Monica lives north of Brisbane with her husband Andreas. Between them they have four beautiful daughters and seven awesome grandchildren.

For Monica's CV and to view more of her work, please visit www.monicabatiste.com.au

Thank you for being you.

I wish you love and peace on your journey.

Monica Batiste

More work by Monica
Yoga for Little Bears

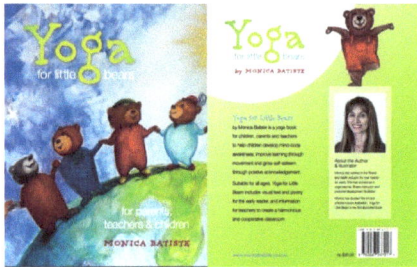

Yoga for little Bears helps children grow emotional intelligence by helping them link movement with emotions. Simple postures such as *Mountain pose* can help a child build the confidence to take a positive stand. *Warrior poses* support a child's courage, and softer postures such as *Resting Butterfly* and *Child's pose* help a child build trust and self-care.

Sometimes children need support in recognizing who they are, and how they feel, in order to socialize more effectively, and to speak up for themselves.

Yoga Bear posture cards (2018)

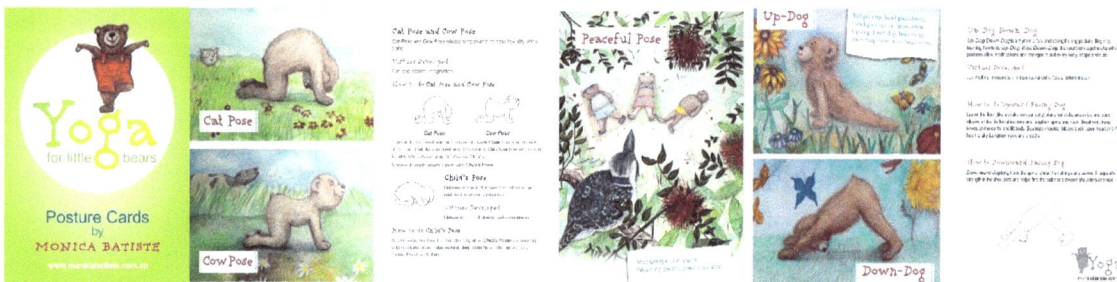

Yoga Bear posture cards are individual cards with yoga poses for children to play with and enjoy. Cards can be selected at random and then performed together in a group, or children can select several cards and create their own practice. There are two sets to choose from; The *Pre Kindy* set is for children who are not yet reading and include the picture plus the poem. This set includes a booklet for adults or older children to read. The *Kids Set* includes a picture of the yoga pose on one side, and text with visual text on the other side for early readers and readers. Both sets are awesome, and will offer support for all ages and abilities.

Simply Yoga and Your Perfect Body (2011)

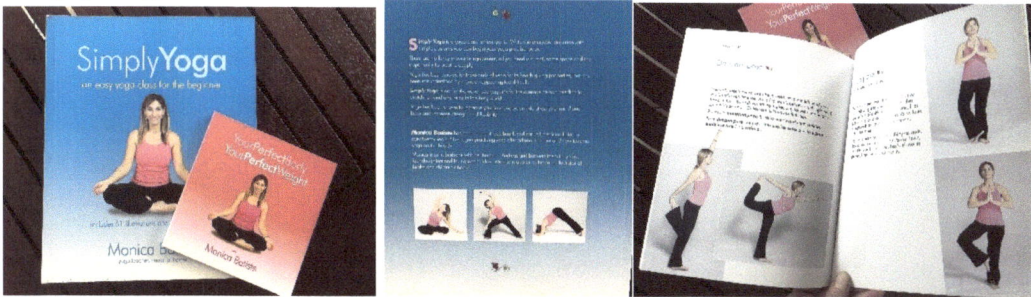

Simply Yoga is a compilation of Monica's beginner yoga class. With 61 illustrations, you will be guided through simple postures and breathing to help you improve in health and relaxation. It begins with easy postures, moves onto stronger options, and finishes with a relaxation. Suitable for the beginner – intermediate.

Simply Yoga is a perfect companion for *'Your Perfect Body'* meditation CD

Your Perfect Body (2011)

Your Perfect Body Your Perfect Weight is a 25-minute meditation to train your conscious and subconscious mind to love eating healthy food (whatever that means for you) and to enjoy exercise (which is unique to you). You will relax deeply during this meditation, learn to appreciate your beautiful body, and allow you to find your perfect health, shape, and freedom. This CD includes two bonus meditations *Heal Your Body colour meditation, a 20* minute meditation on healing and harmonizing your chakras and setting purposeful goals. Plus *Inner Peace* a 10-minute meditation for your quick power naps.

Emotional Freedom Technique; Tap along with Moustache Bear (2015, 2018)

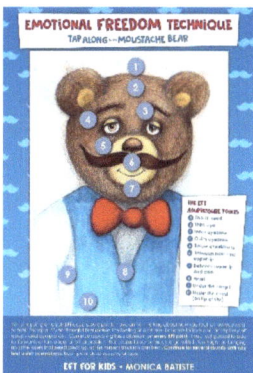

EFT is a simple technique to clear stress from the brain and body. Based on acupressure points, the user 'taps' on points along the face and body whilst 'talking about the problem.' The tapping discharges the negative emotion around the problem and relaxes the brain. This allows the brain to open and allow solutions, as stress shuts the brains ability for problem solving.

Yoga and Virtue pose of the week, *Combining Emotional Intelligence with Yoga* (2015 – 2018)

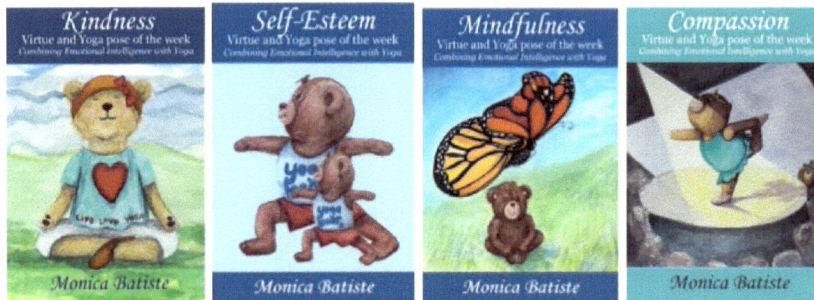

Our innovative program takes the virtues from Emotional Intelligence and combines them with Yoga to build character, strong bodies, and healthy minds.

This is an emotional intelligence program that will boost your child's performance to higher standards, and expand your child's ability to learn.

Combining the science of neuroplasticity on how the brain changes according to thoughts, movement and activities, with the ancient practice of yoga, including mindfulness, deep breathing, focus, strength, and flexibility.

This program has been blended with fun activities, wrapped around the beautiful art of Australian artist and author Monica Batiste.

Each program can be used as a theme for the week, or around topical events.

It is a fun and exciting way of helping children understand their character and virtues.

Each week, a new pose and virtue can be selected, which means, by the end of the school year up to 48 virtues have been grown in children, with a deeper understanding of their mind-body (self-awareness), resilience, confidence, self-regulation and self-esteem.

Benefits for Children
• Overcome the learning difficulties that relate to stress or self-esteem
• Confidence
• Connection to self and others
• Bullies will build empathy
• Timid children will stand up for themselves
• Strength and flexibility

Emotional Intelligence was first recognized by Daniel Goleman, and is considered the most important aspect of development for children to realize their full potential.
The five aspects of Emotional Intelligence are

• Motivation
• Self-esteem
• Social skills
• Self-awareness
• Self-regulation
• Empathy

Features may include
  • A Virtue of the week including cards and printables

- Yoga postures including visual text and printables
- Fun Activities
- Posters and/or colouring in pages for your home or classroom
- Awards or crafty ideas for your children

Virtue and Yoga posture of the week is fun, meaningful and will help your children build a reservoir of emotional intelligence that will benefit the child for his or her entire life.

New programs offered each month

ABC with Yoga Bear and Self-Esteem
PERFECT FOR EARLY READING WRITING AND PAINTING
Interactive Learning

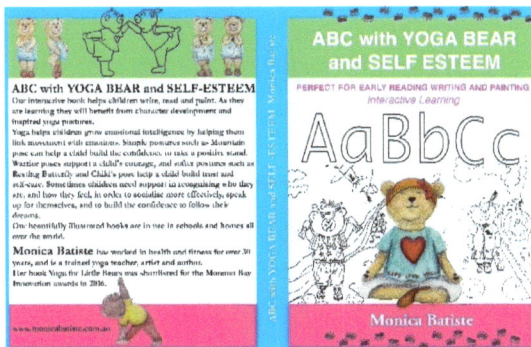

ABC with Yoga Bear to read, write and create your own artistic flair. Perfect for pre and early readers.

References

Arrowsmith Young, B. 2013. The Woman who Changed her Brain. HarperCollins Publishers, Australia.

Dennison, P.E. and Dennison, G.E. 1989. Brain Gym Teachers Edition. Edu-Kinesthetics, USA.

The Brain That Changes Itself. Doidge, N. 2010. Penguin, USA.

Eunson, B. 2011. Communication in the 21st Century (3rd edition). John Wiley & Sons, Milton, Queensland.

Goleman, D. 2006. Emotional Intelligence. (10th anniversary edition) Bantam, New York.

Popov, L. and Popov, D. 1997. The Family Virtues. Plume, New York, USA.

Categories: Health and personal development K-12 PDHPE; Core curriculum; character development. Title: Growing Self-Esteem through Yoga.

ISBN 978-0-6483734-0-7
Published by: Art & Words Publishing, Margate QLD Australia
Author and Illustrator: Monica Batiste; Proofreader: Jane Todd. *Photograph of Monica taken in Berlin with a Berlin Bear of friendship by Gabriela Batiste.*

www.ingramcontent.com/pod-product-compliance
Lightning Source LLC
Chambersburg PA
CBHW060846270326

41933CB00003B/206